WHAT CAN MAKE YOU ILL?

Nester Kadzviti Murira

©N. Murira (2015)

COCKROACH AND FLY

One quiet afternoon Cockroach and Fly met in grandma's kitchen.

'Hello, Roach! What brings you here?' Miss Fly asked as she sat sucking some spilt milk on a table.

'I live here. I clean up. I eat up the leftovers from plates, tables, floors, and anywhere where I can find a morsel of food.

I love dirty kitchens, dirty dishes and dirty floors. I can live there and eat and drink and be very happy.

My kids too can eat and grow fast then join me in the work.' Roach replied.

'Where do you put up your kids, Roach?'

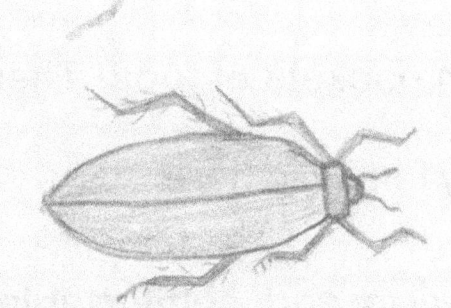

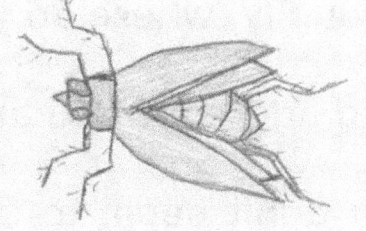

"Oh, there is plenty of room in here! Every crack in the cupboards is home for me and my family.

We can live under mats, under the pots and pans, even in open packets of food! There is plenty of room for me and my family in here.

It is warm and comfortable too!' Roach was almost boasting about where she lives.

What about you Fly, where do you live? You don't seem to have a fixed address? You are flying up and about all the time! You don't seem to settle anywhere?' Roach asked.

'I am kind of busy my friend. I get bored of being in one place and eating the same type of food. I like to look around and see what is interesting, what is delicious, what is nutritious and tasty, so that keeps me very busy.' Fly said proudly.

'What about your kids, where are they and what do they eat while you are here?' Roach asked.

'I lay my eggs anywhere where it is damp and warm and where my kids can easily get food and grow fast. Any heap of warm damp rubbish will do for me! When my kids can fly they can come with me where I go. We sit and eat in many places.' Fly said.

'It must be hard work for you and the kids looking for food then?' Roach felt sorry for Fly.

'Not at all, Roach, I have a wonderful sense of smell. I can tell when and where there is food cooking or when food is being served. I pick the smells then follow the smells and usually when I get there I am not short of surprises. There can be other interesting things too like some sugar, milk and other foods without a strong smell.' Fly said.

'When I am really hungry, anything will do for food. I can sit on children's dirty faces and lick the unwashed food and gravies on the little cheeks, the mucus from the dirty little noses, saliva from the mouths and discharge from eyes. I can lick pus and blood from dirty wounds. When I am really hungry I can even eat a little bit of birds and animals' droppings, human waste, overripe fruit and carcasses.' Fly boasted.

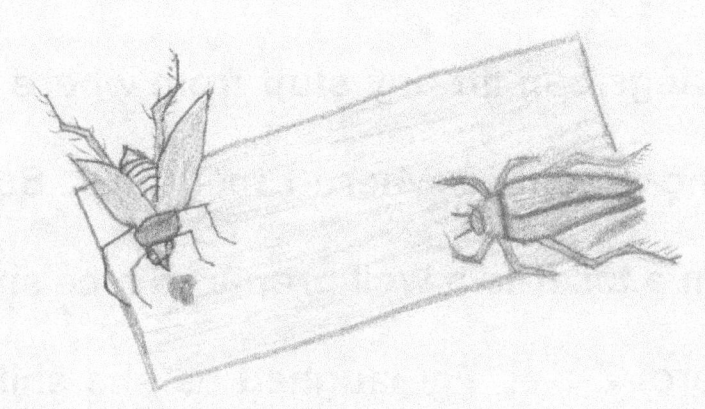

'My life is very interesting, Roach. Fly continued. 'I can eat something really nasty when I am hungry and when I find something nice, I vomit the nasty stuff and eat the nice food. Usually I wash my feet and mouth there and then. My hairy legs can lift any stuff from where I have been eating and take it to where I feed next. So I can carry stuff from a toilet to a well prepared nice smelling dinner anywhere! Z-z-z!' Fly laughed as she shifted to taste jam.

'Well, I also come across hard times. It is not always comfortable in this kitchen.' Roach said.

'Some nights my family and I are sprayed with deadly sprays. We have to go deep into the wooden tiles and skirting and into cracks in cupboards and walls or under the pots and pans to hide. I have taught my kids skills to hide too.' Roach said as Fly listened.

'Sometimes we are forced to leave out in the garden under leaves if the kitchen has been thoroughly cleaned and sprayed with deadly sprays.' Roach explained.

'I have come across sprays too but I fly away fast and escape then come back the next day. What can one do? One has to survive.' Fly said as she shifted to sit on bread crumbs.

Children: Flies and cockroaches carry dirt from one place to the other. Dirt makes one ill.

- Cover your food.

- Clean up the dishes and floors after you have eaten.

- Wash your faces and hands clean.

- Help clean away the rubbish around the home

- Put rubbish in bins or cover it with sand.

- Flies cause sore eyes

- Flies cause a sore tummy.

SNAIL AND MOSQUITO

'Good morning snail! What brings you here everyday? You must be the thirstiest lady in this neighborhood.' Mosquito said in her small annoying voice.

'What are you singing about mosquito? Don't you have happy songs to sing? You are always singing that miserable tune of yours. Anyway, you too are always by this pond. What are you looking for?'Snail asked twiddling her long horns.

'I have a tiny belly my friend. I drink a little water at a time.' Mosquito replied in between tiny sips of water.

'Oh, mosquito, don't I know you well? You are always ready to strike when no one least expects. Tell me the truth.' Snail said.

'Well, snail, my little ones are on that end of the pond hanging on the pond weeds. It is safer for them here because the water is stagnant; I know they will not be swept away by the fast flowing currents of water.' Mosquito said.

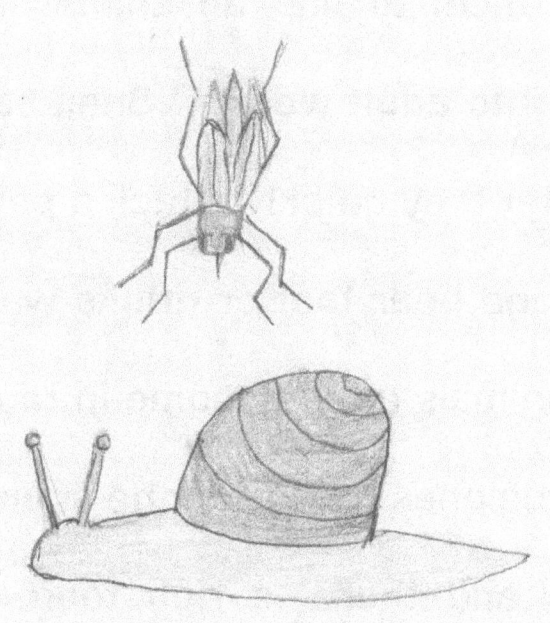

` 'Ah, I am here to help a friend. I carry the little ones for a worm friend, called the bilharzias worm.' Snail smiled. 'I just drop them here and leave them to find an animal in which they can grow into adult worms.' Snail said proudly. 'Once in water they quickly attack a person who gets into the pond bear foot or drinks water from the pond and animals as they come in to drink water. Once the little ones get inside the animal flesh where it is warm and there is rich food, they are free to choose where to live.'

'I did not know you do that, snail? The difference is that I transport malaria worms from one person to the next. It is really a big job for me and my family. When I bite a person, I pick some of the malaria 'falciparum' worms as I take my drink. I then bite the next person and leave some of the worms in the person's blood. The little worms go for the liver and red blood cells of the person. They destroy the liver until the person is very weak and has a high fever or a condition called 'malaria.' When the red blood cells are destroyed the person's eyes and palms turn yellow, what is called 'jaundice.' When the person's red cells are few that is called anemia. If the malaria worms go to the brain then they cause cerebral malaria, a very serious condition. The person with cerebral malaria will need quick attention by the doctor to save his or her life.'

'Really, mosquito?' Snail asked raising her head.

'Of course, snail! Many people know that I am dangerous.'

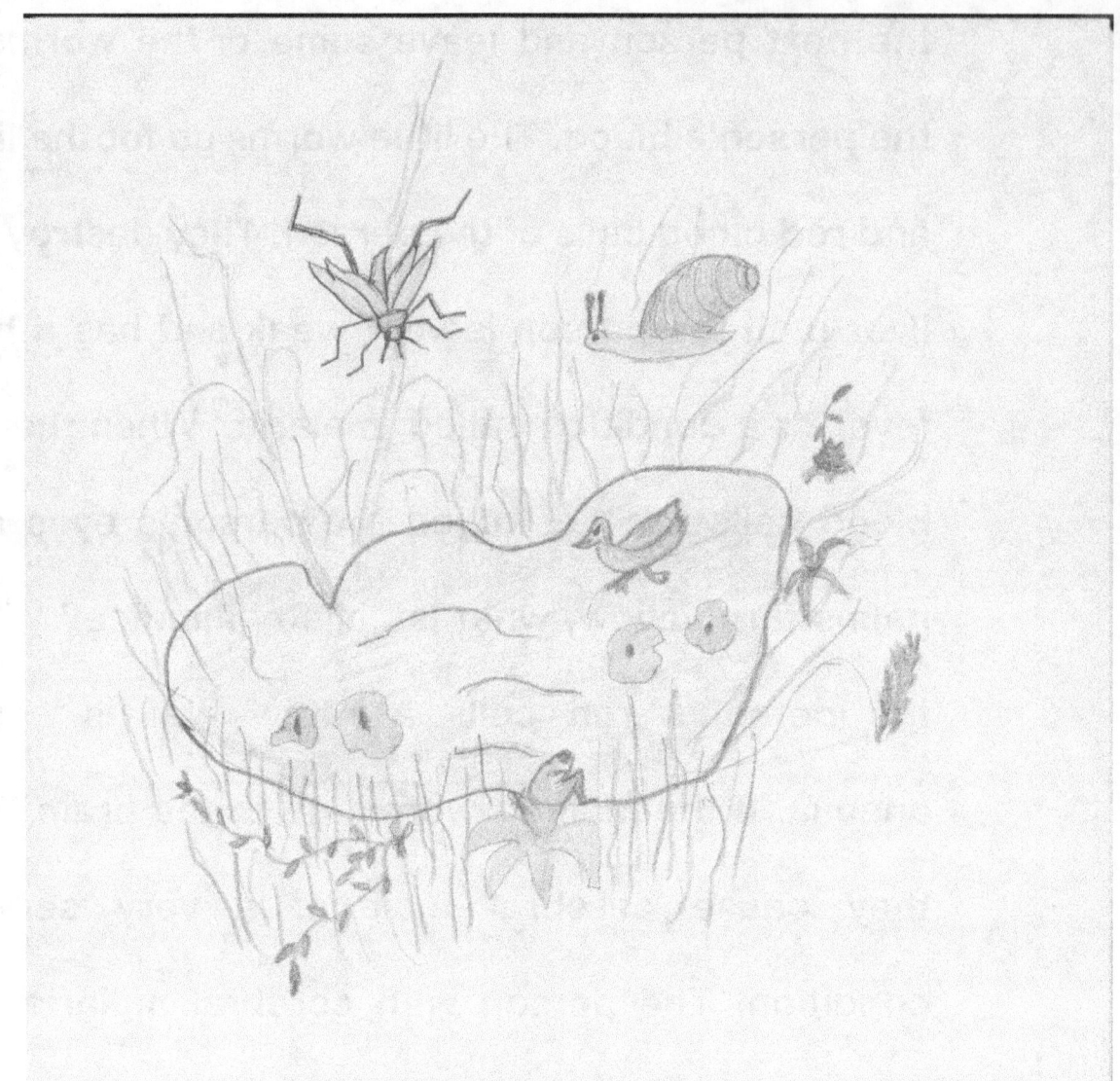

Ah, the bilharzias worms I help settle in the human bladder and bowel and animal muscle. The worms sometimes go to the brain but they cannot be as dangerous as you say you are. Of course they cause some bleeding in the bowel and a few drops of blood in faeces and urine as they try to settle. If a person bleeds for long then they may have anaemia too. You are more dangerous than I thought mosquito! You are actually a lethal danger to people, small as you are!'

'Oh yes, I am, snail. I can infect the whole family in one day by stinging them all and leaving malaria worms in them.' Mosquito sang her evil tune proudly.

'I bite all ages but I am more dangerous to children. They are easy to get too.' Mosquito said.

'Tell me how you pick these worms.' Mosquito asked showing a lot of interest in snail's charity work.

'It is very simple. If infected people with the worms in their bladders or bowels empty their bowels and bladders in an open space or near ponds and streams, the worms are washed into the stream by rain. When I come along with my soft body, the worms easily get inside me where they grow. I release them when they are strong enough to attack a human being or animal.' Snail said.

Prevent mosquito bites:

- Cut grass around the home
- Collect used tins, plastics, bottles and any containers around the home and send them

for re-cycling or bin them for rubbish collectors.

- If you live in rural areas, burn the containers.

- Make holes in the tins and bury them.

- Drain marshes and ponds around the home and cover them with sand.

- Remove weeds and grass from ponds.

- Spray the ponds with paraffin to destroy both the bilharzias worms and mosquito larvae

- Use mosquito repellents such as oils, lotions and creams on your body

- Use mosquito coils and spray insecticides in the homes

- Sleep under medicated mosquito nets all the time. You can ask the health centre near you.

- If you are visiting a malaria area, take medication two weeks before visiting and continue take the medication for two more weeks after visiting a malaria area

- If you have headaches and feel hot and cold, quickly seek treatment at the nearest health centre.

Prevent Bilharzia

- Use toilets for all human waste

- Drain all marshes around

- Spray open sources of water to destroy bilharzias worms (the nearest health centre will assist you).

- Wear rubber shoes if you must work in marshes or need to wade across marshes

- Protect water sources by us of deep wells with a lid or pump.

- Boreholes and where possible piped water are the best sources of drinking water.

- Treat drinking water from open sources with chlorine (the pharmacist will give information on this).

- Boil all drinking water from open sources of water.

- Seek treatment if you notice blood in urine and faeces.

- Snails can be destroyed by sprinkling them with a little salt

THE BIG BLUE FLY

'Zz-zz-zz! I smell some food!'

The big blue fly buzzed making its way to grandma's kitchen.

'Oh, I am so thirsty! I want a nice cool drink.' The big fly licked his dry lips.

'Is that a glass of milk I see on the table? This is my lucky day, isn't it?'

The big blue fly flew to the table.

'Oh, it looks so creamy! I am going to have a good healthy drink! Let me taste it!'

The big blue fly sank his long lips into the glass of cream.

'Mm-mm! This is fresh thick cream! Yummy!

It is so lovely and fresh!

I will take a good drink so that I am full all day!'

I think I will also wash my feet after I have had enough to drink.'

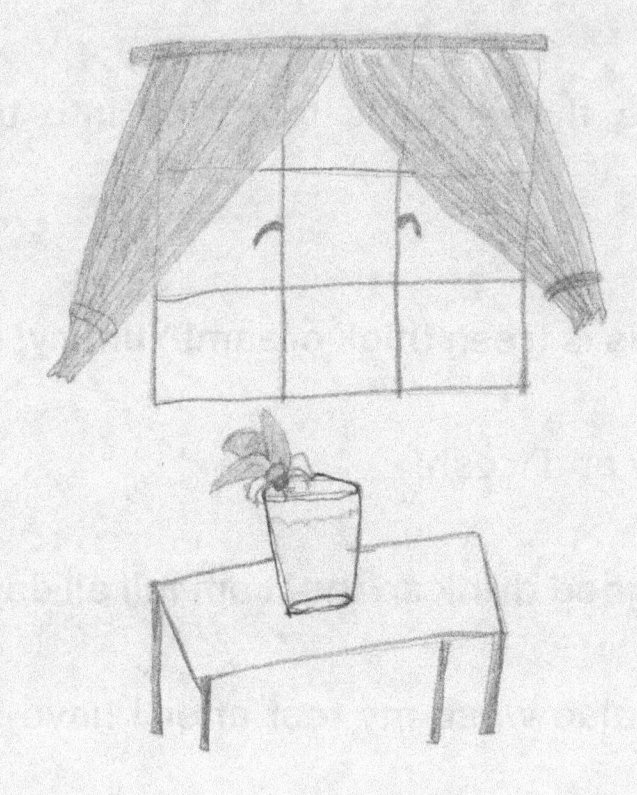

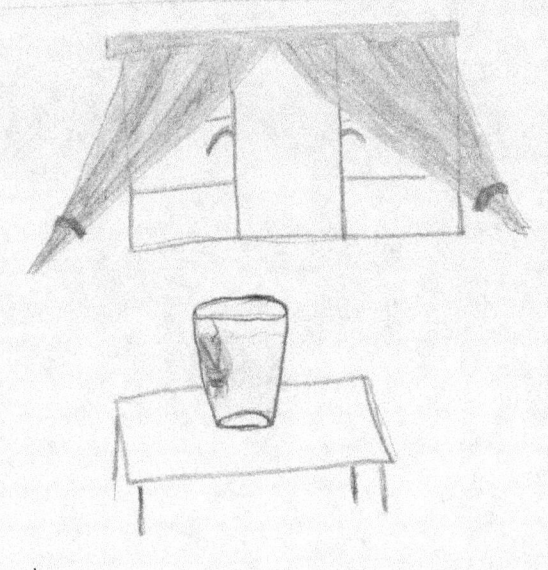

The big fly took a sip of the cream and another and another.

He kept on pushing his feet into the glass as he enjoyed the cream.

Whoops! He fell head first into the glass of cream!

'Oh! Help! Help! Help! Zzz! Zzz.' He tried to shake the cream off his head.

 'It's slippery in here! The glass and the cream are slippery!

Somebody help! I am drowning in the cream!'

The big blue fly buzzed for help but no one came to his help.

The big fly tried to swim out. He went round and round the glass of cream and slipped back and deeper into the glass of cream.

He tried to go up the glass but his legs were slippery.

He tried to fly out but his wings covered in thick cream were so heavy he could not lift them.

He tried to crawl out of the glass but his legs covered in cream were slippery.

His body covered in cream was heavy. He was tired of trying to lift himself out of the cream.

He was so dizzy and sick he vomited into the glass. He fell back into the cream.

He fell asleep in the cream and drowned in the glass of cream.

Children: Always cover milk.

Put milk away in a covered container or in a fridge to keep flies away.

Flies carry germs that make people ill.

WASH AWAY GERMS

Germs are tiny bugs that make people sick.

Germs are found in dust, mud and dirty places.

Some germs stay in parts of our bodies but make us sick when they move to another part of the body .

Germs can be carried onto food by cockroaches and flies.

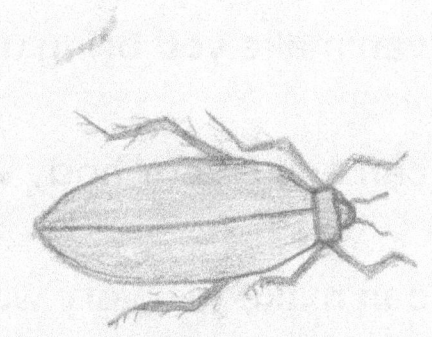

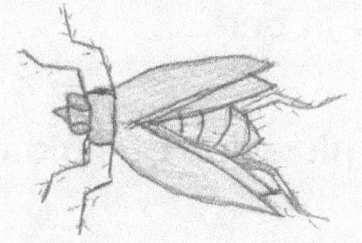

Dirty hands carry germs.

Germs can make your tummy sore.

Germs can make you bring up your food.

Germs can make your body very hot.

Germs can make you very weak.

You cannot play when you are sick.

You must stay in bed.

You must drink a lot of fluids to cool your body and wash away germs.

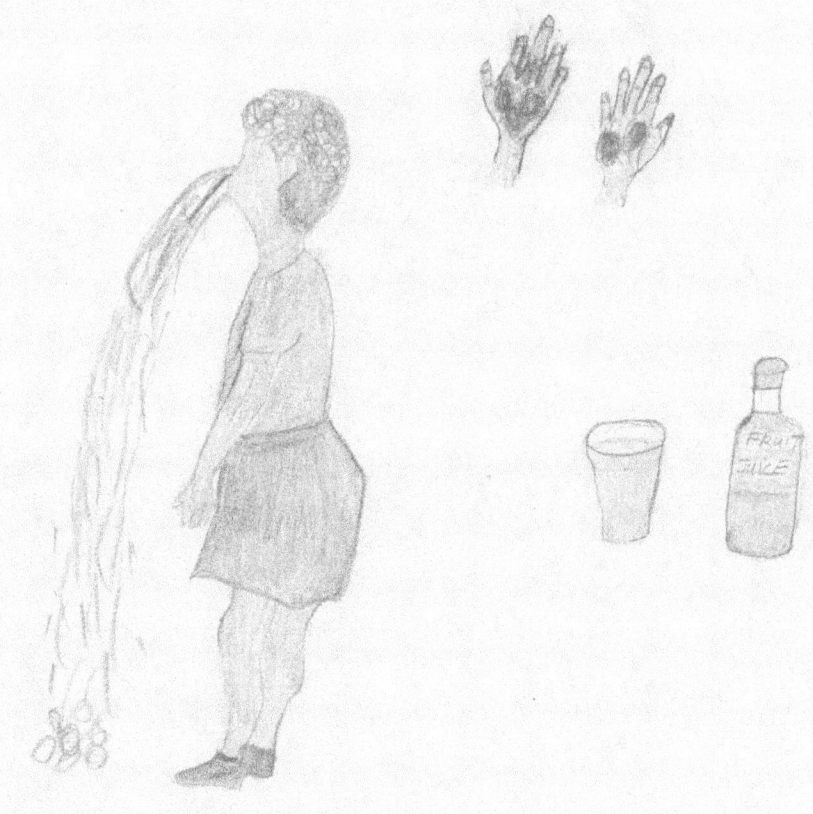

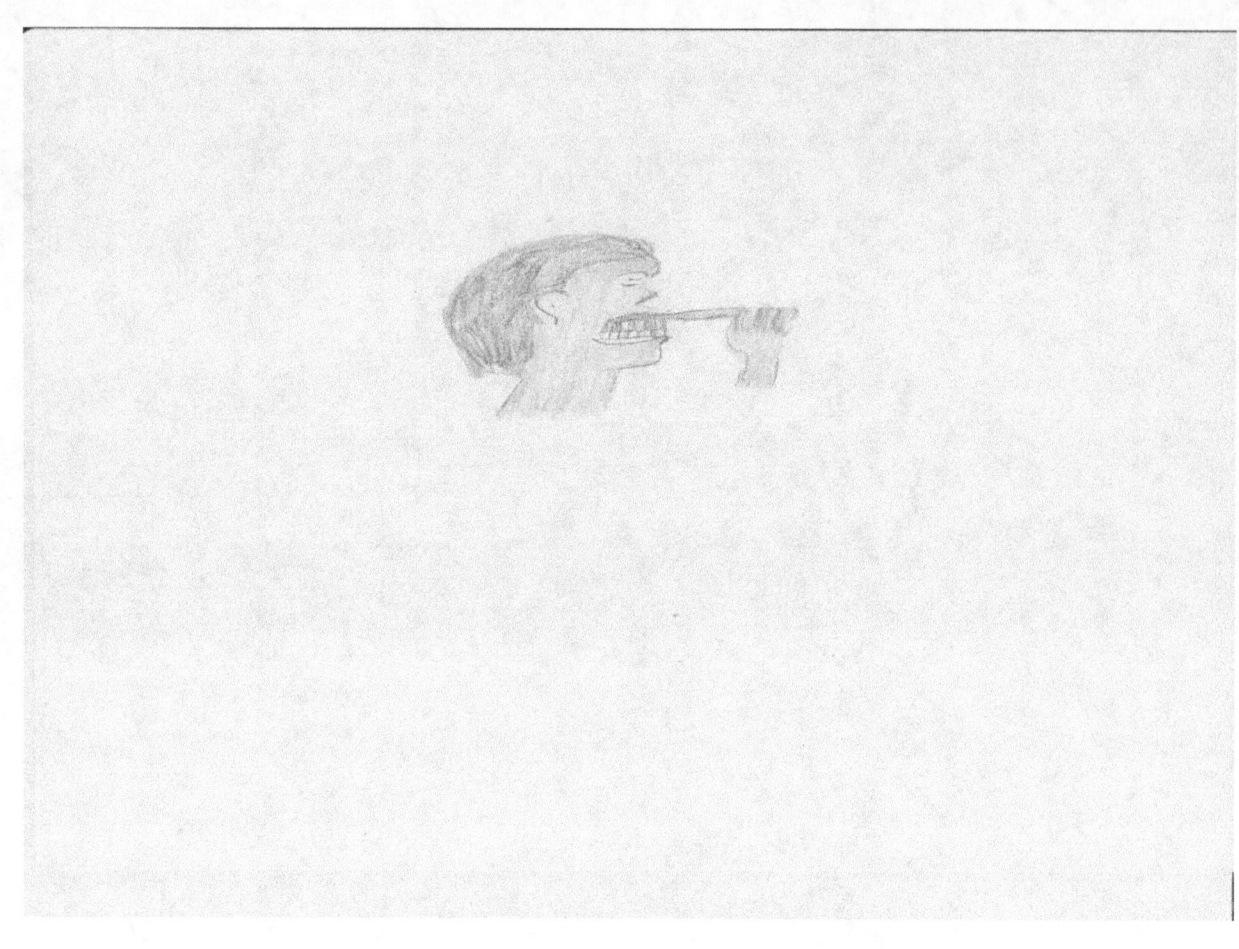

Germs can make holes in your teeth

Brush your teeth after eating Janet!

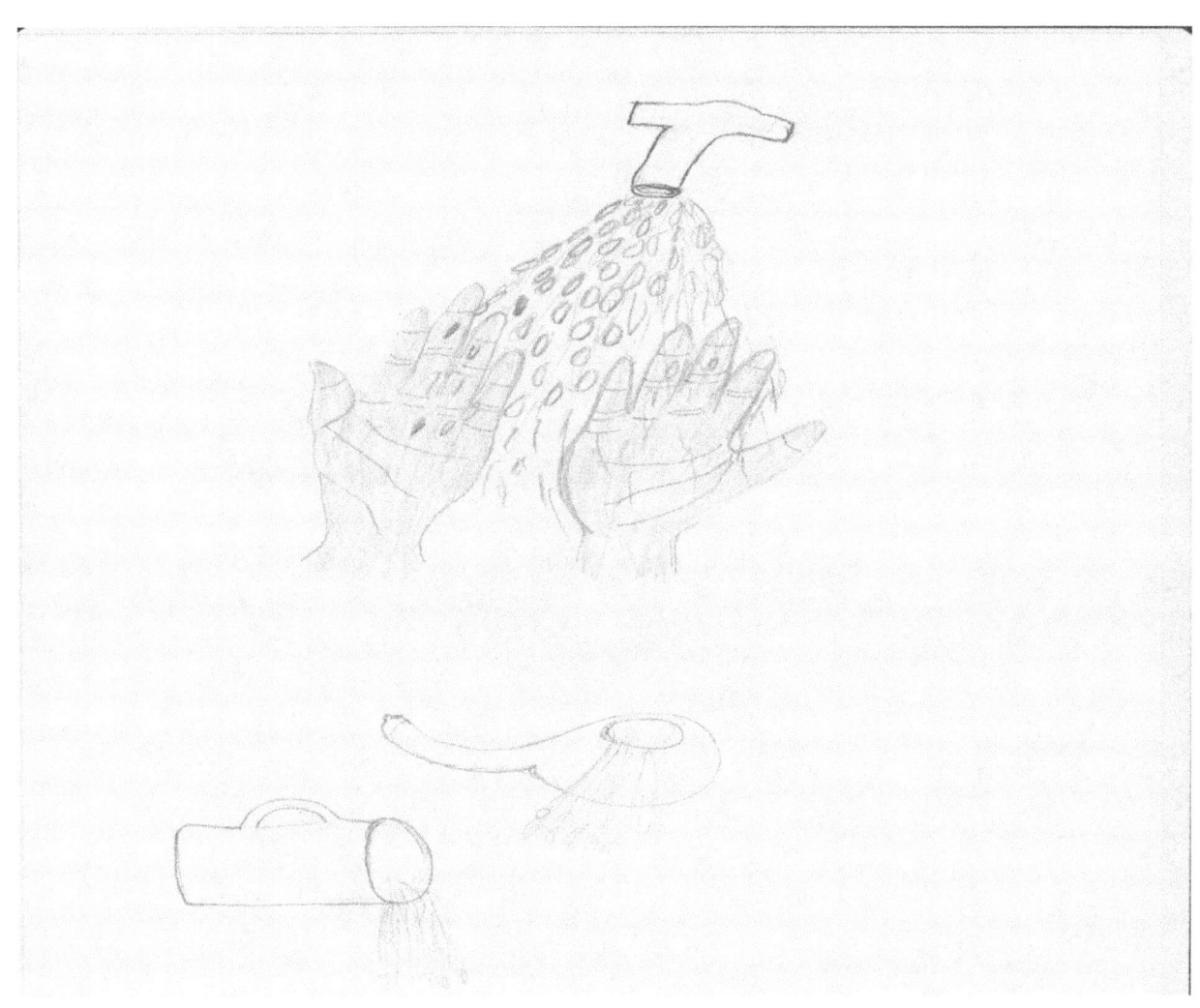

Wash the germs away from your hands Mary!

Wash your hands after using the toilet, John!

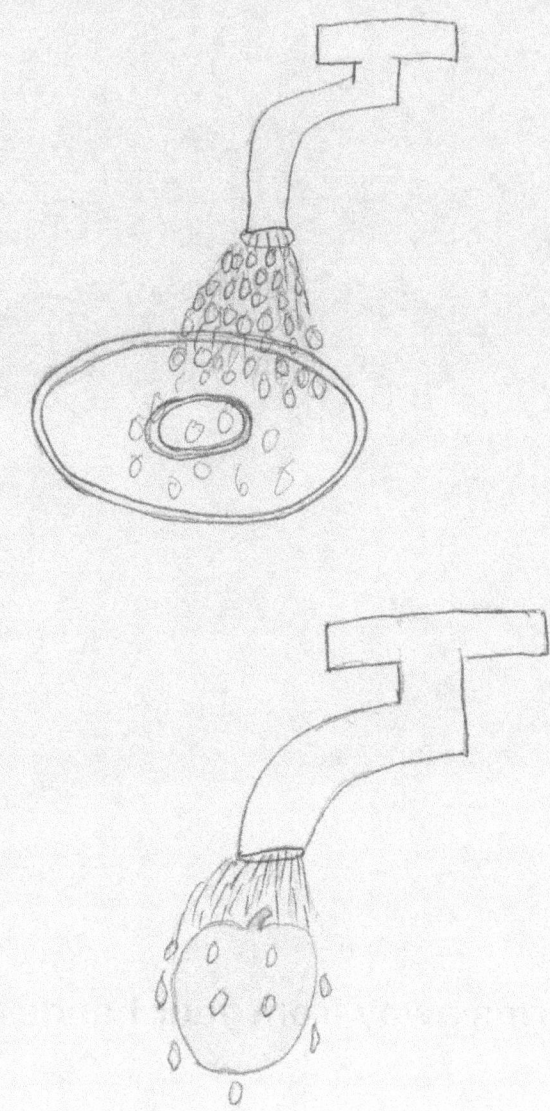

Wash germs from your fruit before you eat, Peter!

Wash your plate clean before you put food, Jane!

Wash your spoon, Teddy!

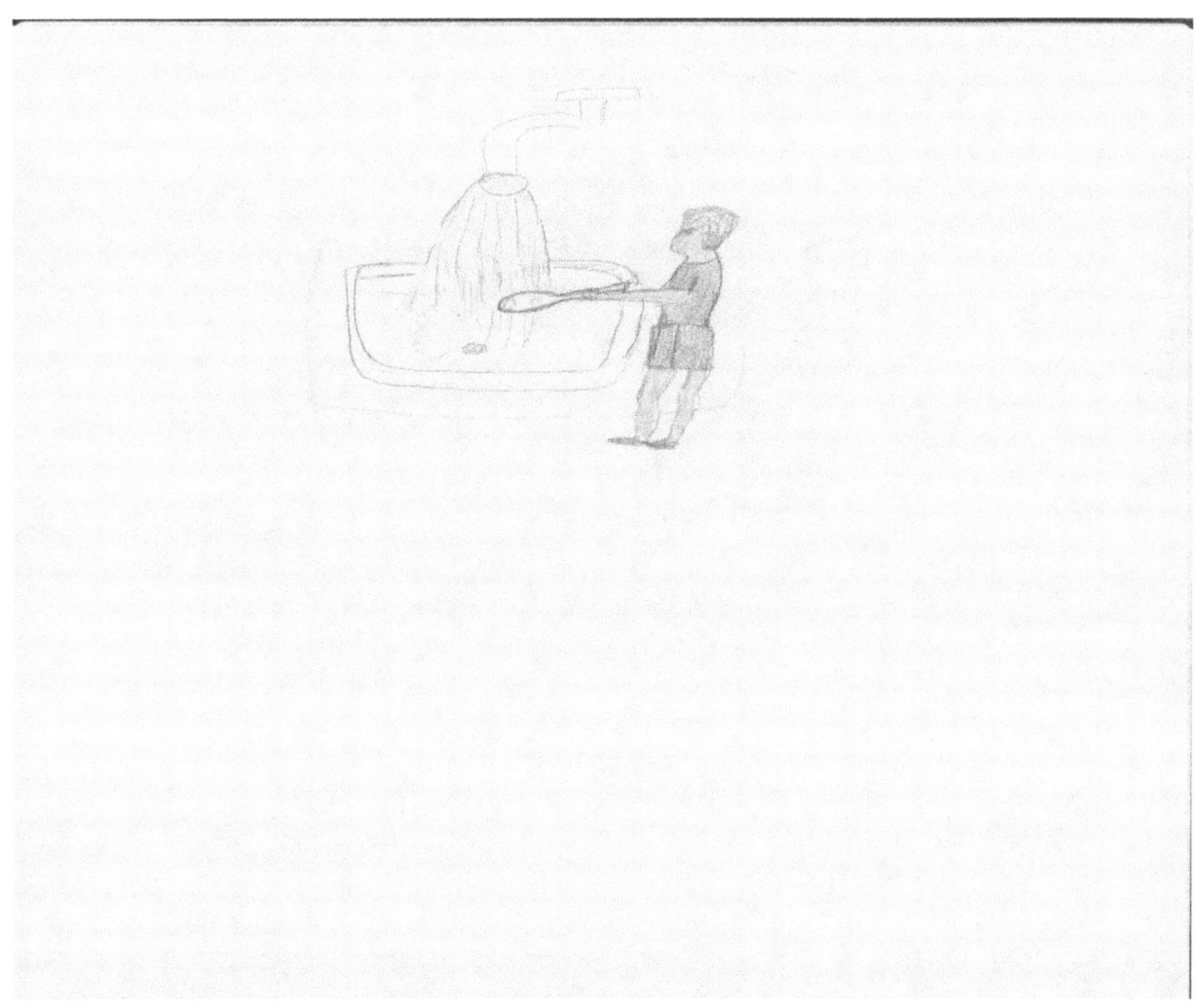

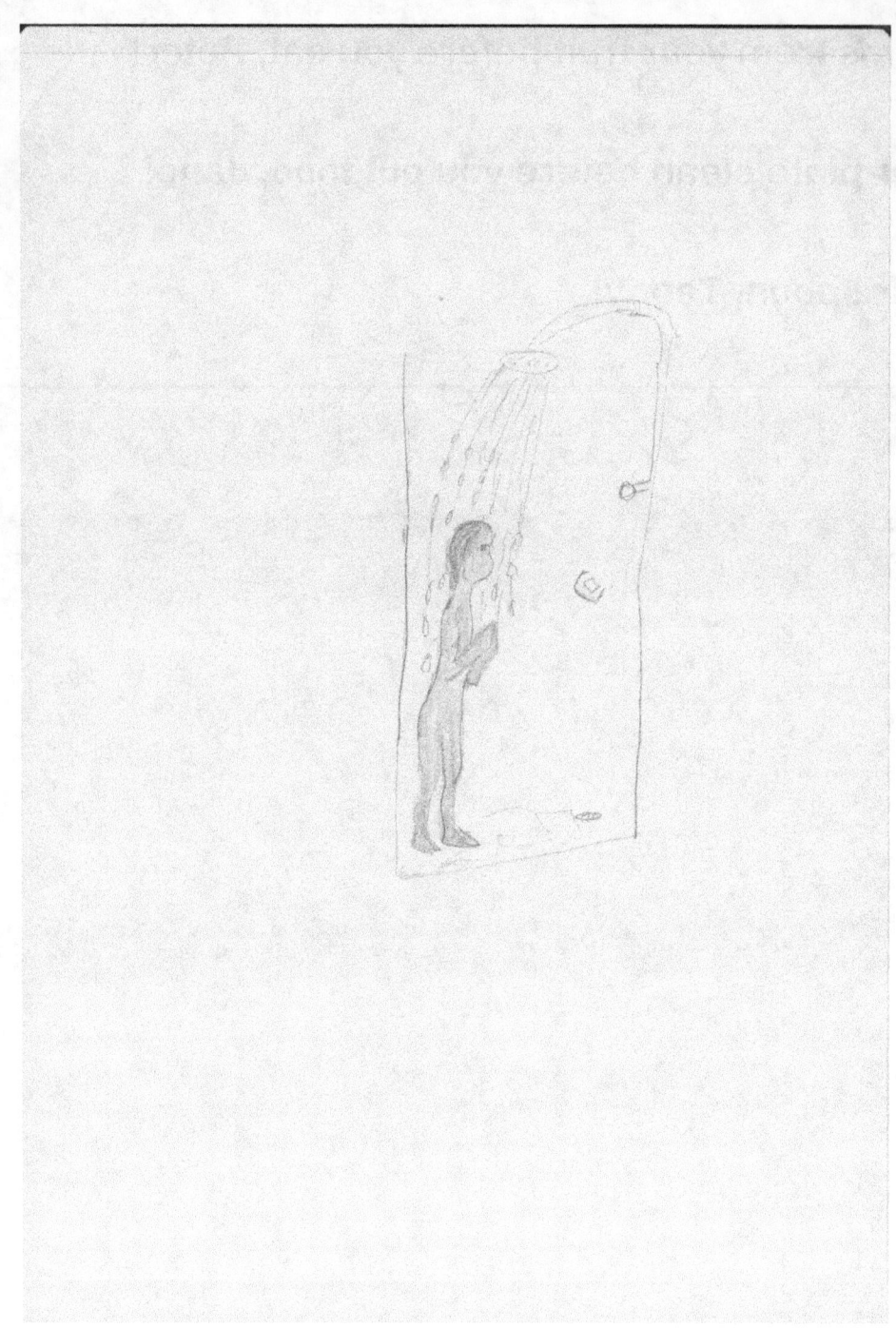

Wash away germs from your body everyday and stay healthy!

LITTLE MOTH

One cold evening, a little grey moth saw a bright candle light.

'I will fly round the candle to get warm.' Little moth said.

Little moth flew round and round the candle once, twice, three times!

'I feel warm now but I like to stay near the light and stay warm!' Little moth said.

'It is fun going round the candle!' Little moth smiled.

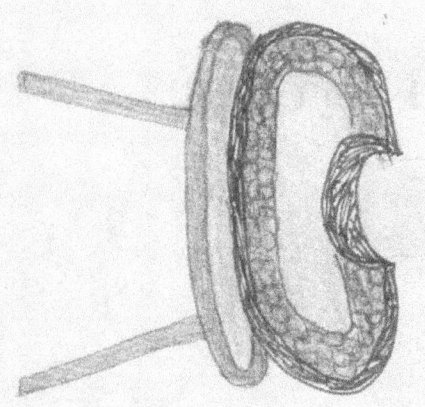

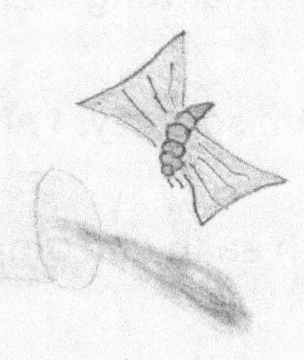

'Round and round here I go! Round and round here I go! Round and round here I go until I get warmer!' Sang little moth.

'Oh, oh, I am getting dizzy!' Little moth giggled.

'Dizzy! I am so dizzy! I am so dizzy I can't stop!'

Little moth sang and giggled.

'Wow! Wow! Wow! I am dizzy!

Hoopsy daisy! Oh, hot candle wax!'

'Oh-o-o-o! I fell on hot candle wax! I am burning up! I am burning up.' Little moth cried.

Little moth was stuck in hot candle wax. Her wings caught fire.

'Help, my wings caught fire! I am burning!' She cried for help but no one heard and she was burnt to ashes.

Boys and girls:

- Don't play near fire. Your clothes may catch fire.

- Fire can hurt you and other people around.

- Fire burns grass,trees and homes.

- Fire hurts animals too.

Prevent fires:

- Don't play with fire, cigarette lighter or matches.

- Keep away from hot stoves and boiling water. Burns are very painful and can make you very ill.

Fluids and your health

A healthy body needs fluids to stay healthy.

 Why does the body need fluids?

The body needs fluids to make blood and keep blood flowing to all pats of the body. Blood is life. Blood carries oxygen (air), food and protection to all parts of the body especially the parts that keep us alive (vital organs) which are the heart, the lungs, the brain, kidneys and the liver.

Every part of your body needs a good blood supply to keep it healthy.

Your body needs fluids to digest food.

You need fluids to have normal bowel movements and prevent constipation (hard faeces)

Fluids make mucus in the nose, throat and lungs.

Mucus stops germs and dust from getting in the chest.

Germs and dust cause coughs and pain in the chest.

Fluids wash away dirt and poisons from the body.

You need fluids to wash away poisons from the body.

Fluids prevent disease of the bladder and kidneys.

The body needs fluids to make tears and saliva.

Fluids cool the body and prevent fevers.

Fluid Loss

The body looses fluid through sweat.

Dress lightly in hot weather.

Drink plenty of fluids in hot weather.

Fluid is lost through bowel movements, urine, vomiting, bleeding, yawning, talking, and singing. Replace fluids lost to keep healthy.

The body needs more fluid if one is active, sweating, sick and when the weather is hot.

Fluids and children

Children need plenty of fluids to prevent the skin from drying up.

When you don't have enough fluids in your body, your skin is hot, your tongue is dry and furry and you pass little dark urine.

If you have a sore tummy and you are vomiting, you must drink lots of fluids to replace the fluids you are loosing.

Drink fluids after every meal and when it is hot.

Carry bottles of water and other nourishing fluids (fruit juice) when going to school and when travelling.

www.ingramcontent.com/pod-product-compliance
Lightning Source LLC
Chambersburg PA
CBHW080615180526
45168CB00007B/2923

9 781517 183790